WEIGHT LOSS AFTER PREGNANCY COOKBOOK

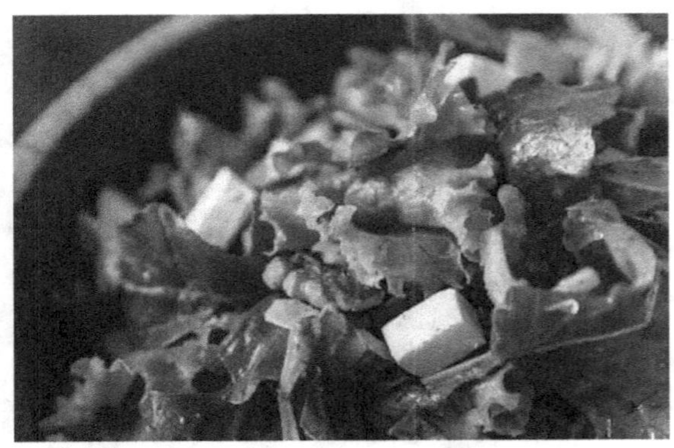

DR. JESSICA SMITH

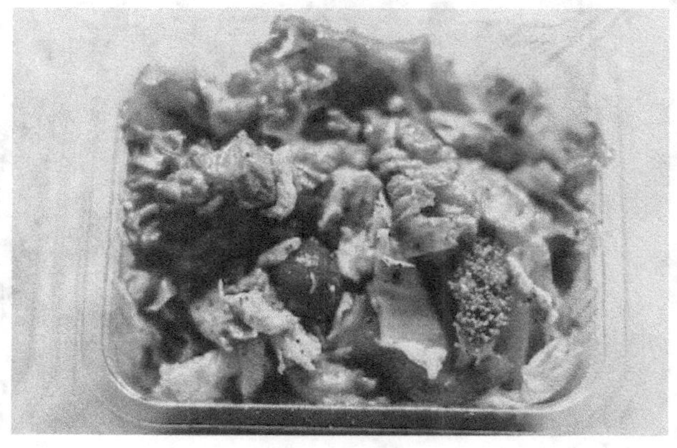

TABLE OF CONTENTS

CHAPTER ONE

How to Use this Cookbook

Losing weight after pregnancy requires a balanced approach that combines healthy eating with regular physical activity.

The "Weight Loss After Pregnancy Cookbook" can be a valuable tool to support your journey to a healthier and more sustainable weight.

Here's a guide on how to use the cookbook effectively:

Consult with Your Healthcare Provider:

Before making any significant changes to your diet, especially post-pregnancy, it's crucial to consult with your healthcare provider. They can provide personalized advice based on your health, nutritional needs, and any specific considerations related to your postpartum recovery.

Understand Nutritional Needs:

The cookbook likely emphasizes nutrient-dense, balanced meals. Pay attention to the recommended portion sizes and ensure you're getting a variety of nutrients, including essential vitamins and minerals. Aim for a well-rounded diet that supports both your weight loss goals and your overall well-being.

Meal Planning:

Plan your meals in advance based on the recipes provided in the cookbook. This can help you make healthier food choices and reduce the likelihood of opting for less nutritious options when you're pressed for time. Consider planning for a week at a time and create a shopping list accordingly.

Balanced Macronutrients:

The cookbook may offer a mix of macronutrients (carbohydrates, proteins, and fats) to keep you satisfied and provide sustained energy. Pay attention to the balance and choose recipes that align with your nutritional goals.

Incorporate Regular Physical Activity:

While the cookbook focuses on nutrition, remember that weight loss is a holistic journey. Combine healthy eating with regular physical activity. Consult with your healthcare provider to determine suitable exercises based on your postpartum recovery.

Hydration: Staying hydrated is crucial for overall health and can support weight loss. Water is essential, and you can also incorporate hydrating foods like fruits and vegetables from the cookbook.

Listen to Your Body:

Pay attention to your body's hunger and fullness cues. The cookbook's recipes may help you develop a healthier relationship with food. Eat mindfully, savoring each bite, and stop when you're satisfied.

Be Patient and Realistic:

Weight loss after pregnancy is a gradual process. Be patient with yourself, and set realistic goals. The cookbook likely provides sustainable recipes to support long-term success rather than quick fixes.

Involve Your Support System:

Share your journey with friends, family, or other new moms. A supportive community can provide encouragement, share tips, and make the process more enjoyable.

Track Progress: Keep a record of your meals, physical activity, and how you feel. Tracking your progress can help you stay motivated and identify what works best for you.

Remember, every postpartum journey is unique, and what works for one person may not work for another.

Use the cookbook as a resource to inspire and guide you toward making healthier choices as you work towards your weight loss goals.

If you have any concerns or questions, consult with your healthcare provider for personalized advice.

Understanding Weight Loss after Pregnancy

Weight loss after pregnancy is a multifaceted journey that demands a nuanced understanding of the body's unique postpartum needs.

While shedding excess weight is a common goal, it's essential to approach this process with patience, empathy, and a focus on holistic well-being. The body undergoes profound changes during pregnancy, and the postpartum period requires careful attention to both physical and emotional aspects.

A key consideration is establishing a realistic timeline for weight loss, acknowledging that the body needs time to recover.

A balanced and nutrient-rich diet, coupled with regular physical activity, forms the foundation of a healthy weight loss strategy.

The "Weight Loss After Pregnancy Cookbook" can serve as a valuable guide, offering recipes tailored to postpartum nutritional needs.

Understanding that weight loss is not a one-size-fits-all journey is crucial.

Factors such as breastfeeding, hormonal fluctuations, and individual metabolic rates vary among women.

It's important to prioritize overall health, focusing on nourishing foods that provide energy and support recovery.

Moreover, postpartum weight loss is an emotional and psychological process.

Embracing self-compassion, seeking support, and fostering a positive body image contribute significantly to a successful and sustainable weight loss journey.

In navigating weight loss after pregnancy, a holistic approach that integrates physical and emotional well-being is paramount, paving the way for a healthier, happier postpartum experience.

Principles of Weight Loss after Pregnancy

The principles of weight loss after pregnancy revolve around a balanced, gradual, and holistic approach that prioritizes both physical health and emotional well-being.

Firstly, understanding the unique needs of the postpartum body is essential. The recovery process demands a thoughtful combination of nutrient-dense foods that aid healing and support energy levels.

The "Weight Loss After Pregnancy Cookbook" adheres to these principles by offering recipes that strike a harmonious balance between nourishment and weight management.

Secondly, portion control and mindful eating play pivotal roles.

The cookbook likely emphasizes portion sizes that satisfy hunger while promoting weight loss. Learning to listen to one's body signals, distinguishing between emgotional and physical hunger, forms a cornerstone of postpartum weight loss principles.

Incorporating regular physical activity aligns with these principles, fostering a healthy metabolism and aiding in weight management.

However, the exercise routine should be tailored to individual postpartum recovery, ensuring a gradual progression.

Moreover, recognizing that postpartum weight loss is a journey unique to each woman is crucial. Setting realistic goals, celebrating small victories, and cultivating a positive relationship with one's body contribute to sustainable weight loss principles.

Ultimately, these principles underscore the importance of patience, self-compassion, and a comprehensive approach that embraces the intricate balance of physical and emotional aspects during the postpartum period.

Benefits of Weight Loss after Pregnancy

Weight loss after pregnancy offers a myriad of benefits that extend beyond physical appearance, encompassing both the physical and emotional dimensions of a woman's well-being. Firstly, shedding excess weight reduces the risk of long-term health issues such as diabetes and heart disease, supporting overall cardiovascular health.

Postpartum weight loss contributes to increased energy levels and stamina, essential for navigating the demands of motherhood.

This newfound vitality promotes an active lifestyle, positively impacting mental health and fostering a sense of accomplishment.

The "Weight Loss After Pregnancy Cookbook" likely aids in this process by providing recipes that optimize nutritional intake for sustained energy.

Moreover, achieving a healthy weight after childbirth often enhances self-esteem and body confidence.

Embracing one's postpartum body and feeling comfortable in one's skin fosters a positive body image, promoting mental well-being.

Weight loss after pregnancy can also positively impact hormonal balance, potentially aiding in the regulation of menstrual cycles and improving fertility for those considering future pregnancies.

Beyond physical health, the emotional benefits of postpartum weight loss are significant.

It can reduce feelings of stress and anxiety, contributing to an improved overall mood and mental resilience.

Ultimately, the holistic advantages of weight loss after pregnancy encompass physical health, emotional well-being, and the empowerment to navigate the joys and challenges of motherhood with confidence.

Tips for Weight Loss after Pregnancy

Embarking on a weight loss journey after pregnancy requires a thoughtful and holistic approach. First and foremost, consult with your healthcare provider to establish a safe and personalized plan tailored to your postpartum recovery. Here are some valuable tips to guide you through the process:

Nutrient-Rich Diet: Focus on a well-balanced, nutrient-dense diet. The "Weight Loss After Pregnancy Cookbook" can be a valuable resource, providing recipes rich in vitamins, minerals, and essential nutrients crucial for postpartum recovery.

Hydration is Key: Adequate water intake supports overall health and aids in weight loss. Stay hydrated to boost energy levels and assist in metabolism.

Mindful Eating: Practice mindful eating by paying attention to hunger and fullness cues. Savor each bite, and be aware of emotional triggers that may lead to overeating.

Regular Physical Activity: Incorporate gentle exercises into your routine as per your healthcare provider's recommendations. Gradual reintroduction of physical activity supports weight loss and overall well-being.

Adequate Sleep: Prioritize sufficient and quality sleep. Lack of sleep can impact metabolism and increase cravings for unhealthy foods.

Set Realistic Goals: Establish achievable, realistic weight loss goals. Celebrate small victories, and understand that postpartum weight loss is a gradual process.

Effective weight loss after pregnancy involves adopting sensible guidelines that prioritize health, sustainability, and the unique needs of postpartum recovery.

Begin by obtaining clearance from your healthcare provider to embark on a weight loss journey. Once approved, consider the following guidelines:

Gradual Approach: Aim for a gradual weight loss of about 1-2 pounds per week. This approach is both safe and sustainable, preventing drastic measures that may compromise your health or hinder milk supply if breastfeeding.

Nutrient-Dense Foods: Prioritize nutrient-dense foods, including whole grains, lean proteins, fruits, and vegetables. The "Weight Loss After Pregnancy Cookbook" can guide you in creating delicious, balanced meals that nourish both you and your baby.

Portion Control: Be mindful of portion sizes to avoid overeating. Listen to your body's hunger and fullness cues, and avoid restrictive diets that may compromise energy levels.

Hydration: Stay well-hydrated, as adequate water intake is crucial for overall health and can aid in weight loss.

Incorporate Physical Activity: Gradually reintroduce physical activity as per your healthcare provider's recommendations. Include a mix of aerobic exercises, strength training, and flexibility exercises to enhance overall fitness.

Prioritize Self-Care: Prioritize self-care to manage stress, which can impact weight loss. Incorporate activities you enjoy, practice mindfulness, and ensure adequate sleep.

Breastfeeding Considerations: If breastfeeding, be mindful of caloric needs and avoid extreme calorie deficits. Focus on a balanced diet that supports both weight loss and milk production. .

Social Support: Engage with a supportive community, whether it's other new moms, friends, or family. Share your experiences, seek advice, and celebrate successes together.

Self-Compassion: Be kind to yourself. Recognize the challenges of postpartum life and embrace the changes in your body with self-compassion.

CHAPTER TWO

Weight Loss after Pregnancy Recipes

1: Grilled Lemon Herb Salmon

Ingredients:

- ➢ 4 salmon fillets
- ➢ 2 tablespoons olive oil
- ➢ 1 lemon (juiced)
- ➢ Fresh herbs (such as dill or parsley)
- ➢ Salt and pepper to taste
- ➢ Instructions:
- ➢ Preheat the grill.
- ➢ In a bowl, mix olive oil, lemon juice, fresh herbs, salt, and pepper.
- ➢ Brush the salmon fillets with the mixture.
- ➢ Grill for 4-5 minutes per side until the salmon is cooked through.

Health Benefits:

- ➢ Salmon provides omega-3 fatty acids for heart health.
- ➢ Olive oil offers healthy fats.

➢ Fresh herbs add flavor without additional calories.

Preparation Time: 15 minutes

2: Quinoa and Roasted Vegetable Bowl

Ingredients:

➢ 1 cup quinoa (cooked)

➢ Assorted vegetables (bell peppers, zucchini, cherry tomatoes)

➢ 2 tablespoons balsamic vinegar

➢ 1 tablespoon olive oil

➢ Salt and pepper to taste

Instructions:

➢ Preheat the oven to 400°F (200°C).

➢ Toss vegetables with olive oil, balsamic vinegar, salt, and pepper.

➢ Roast for 20-25 minutes.

➢ Serve over a bed of cooked quinoa.

Health Benefits:

➢ Quinoa provides protein and fiber.

➢ Vegetables offer vitamins and antioxidants.

➢ Balsamic vinegar adds flavor without extra calories.

Preparation Time: 30 minutes

3: Greek Yogurt Parfait

Ingredients:

- 1 cup Greek yogurt
- 1/2 cup mixed berries
- 2 tablespoons granola
- 1 tablespoon honey

Instructions:

- In a glass, layer Greek yogurt, mixed berries, and granola.
- Drizzle honey on top.
- Repeat the layers.
- Enjoy as a nutrient-rich breakfast or snack.

Health Benefits:

- Greek yogurt provides protein.
- Berries offer antioxidants.
- Granola adds crunch and fiber.

Preparation Time: 5 minutes

4: Turkey and Vegetable Stir-Fry

Ingredients:

- 1 pound lean ground turkey
- Assorted vegetables (broccoli, bell peppers, snap peas)
- 2 tablespoons low-sodium soy sauce
- 1 tablespoon sesame oil
- 1 teaspoon ginger (minced)
- 2 cloves garlic (minced)

Instructions:

- In a wok or skillet, brown ground turkey.
- Add vegetables, soy sauce, sesame oil, ginger, and garlic.
- Stir-fry until vegetables are tender.
- Serve over brown rice or cauliflower rice.

Health Benefits:

- Lean turkey provides protein.
- Colorful vegetables offer vitamins.
- Low-sodium soy sauce adds flavor.

Preparation Time: 25 minutes

5: Spinach and Feta Stuffed Chicken Breast

Ingredients:

- 4 boneless, skinless chicken breasts
- 2 cups fresh spinach
- 1/2 cup feta cheese (crumbled)
- 2 tablespoons olive oil
- Salt and pepper to taste

Instructions:

- Preheat the oven to 375°F (190°C).
- Butterfly the chicken breasts.
- Sauté spinach in olive oil until wilted.
- Stuff each chicken breast with spinach and feta.
- Season with salt and pepper.
- Bake for 25-30 minutes or until chicken is cooked through.

Health Benefits:

- Chicken is a lean source of protein.
- Spinach provides iron and vitamins.
- Feta adds flavor without excessive calories.

Preparation Time: 40 minutes

6: Lentil and Vegetable Soup

Ingredients:

- 1 cup lentils (rinsed and drained)
- Assorted vegetables (carrots, celery, onion)
- 4 cups low-sodium vegetable broth
- 1 teaspoon cumin
- 1 teaspoon paprika
- Salt and pepper to taste

Instructions:

- In a pot, sauté vegetables until softened.
- Add lentils, vegetable broth, cumin, paprika, salt, and pepper.
- Simmer for 25-30 minutes or until lentils are tender.

Health Benefits:

- Lentils provide protein and fiber.
- Vegetables offer vitamins and minerals.
- A hearty, low-calorie soup option.

Preparation Time: 40 minutes

7: Baked Egg and Vegetable Cups

Ingredients:

- 6 eggs
- Assorted vegetables (bell peppers, spinach, cherry tomatoes)
- 1/4 cup feta cheese (optional)
- Salt and pepper to taste

Instructions:

- Preheat the oven to 375°F (190°C).
- Grease a muffin tin.
- Crack an egg into each muffin cup.
- Add chopped vegetables and sprinkle with feta.
- Bake for 15-20 minutes or until eggs are set.

Health Benefits:

- Eggs provide protein.
- Vegetables offer vitamins and fiber.
- A quick and easy breakfast option.

Preparation Time: 20 minutes

8: Sweet Potato and Black Bean Quesadillas

Ingredients:

- 2 large sweet potatoes (cooked and mashed)
- 1 can black beans (drained and rinsed)
- Whole-grain tortillas
- 1 cup shredded cheese (low-fat)
- 1 teaspoon cumin
- 1 teaspoon chili powder

Instructions:

- In a bowl, mix mashed sweet potatoes, black beans, cumin, and chili powder.
- Spread the mixture on a tortilla and sprinkle with cheese.
- Top with another tortilla.
- Cook on a skillet until cheese is melted and tortillas are crispy.

Health Benefits:

- Sweet potatoes offer vitamins and fiber.
- Black beans provide protein and fiber.
- Whole-grain tortillas add complex carbohydrates.

Preparation Time: 30 minutes

9: Avocado and Chickpea Salad

Ingredients:

- ➤ 2 avocados (diced)
- ➤ 1 can chickpeas (drained and rinsed)
- ➤ Cherry tomatoes (halved)
- ➤ 1/4 cup red onion (finely chopped)
- ➤ 2 tablespoons cilantro (chopped)
- ➤ Lime juice for dressing

Instructions:

- ➤ In a bowl, combine diced avocados, chickpeas, cherry tomatoes, red onion, and cilantro.
- ➤ Drizzle with lime juice and toss gently.
- ➤ Serve as a refreshing salad or side dish.

Health Benefits:

- ➤ Avocados offer healthy fats.
- ➤ Chickpeas provide protein and fiber.
- ➤ A light and nutritious salad option.

Preparation Time: 15 minutes

10: Zucchini Noodles with Pesto

Ingredients:

> - 4 medium zucchinis (spiralized into noodles)
> - 1/2 cup cherry tomatoes (halved)
> - 1/4 cup pine nuts
> - 1 cup fresh basil leaves
> - 1/4 cup Parmesan cheese (grated)
> - 2 cloves garlic
> - 1/2 cup olive oil
> - Salt and pepper to taste

Instructions:

> - In a blender, combine basil, pine nuts, garlic, and Parmesan.
> - While blending, slowly add olive oil until smooth.
> - Toss zucchini noodles with cherry tomatoes and pesto.
> - Season with salt and pepper.

Health Benefits:

> - Zucchini provides a low-calorie alternative to pasta.
> - Pesto offers vibrant flavors without excess calories.

➢ A light and satisfying option for lunch or dinner.

Preparation Time: 20 minutes

11: Cucumber and Salmon Sushi Rolls

Ingredients:

- ➢ Nori sheets
- ➢ 2 cups cauliflower rice (cooked)
- ➢ Smoked salmon slices
- ➢ Cucumber strips
- ➢ Avocado slices
- ➢ Low-sodium soy sauce for dipping

Instructions:

- ➢ Place a nori sheet on a bamboo sushi rolling mat.
- ➢ Spread a layer of cauliflower rice on the nori.
- ➢ Arrange smoked salmon, cucumber, and avocado along one edge.
- ➢ Roll tightly using the bamboo mat.
- ➢ Slice into bite-sized pieces and serve with soy sauce.

Health Benefits:

- ➢ Cauliflower rice reduces carb content.
- ➢ Salmon provides omega-3 fatty acids.

> ➢ A nutritious and creative sushi alternative.

Preparation Time: 25 minutes

12: Blueberry Almond Smoothie Bowl

Ingredients:

- ➢ 1 cup frozen blueberries
- ➢ 1 banana
- ➢ 1/2 cup almond milk
- ➢ 1/4 cup Greek yogurt
- ➢ Toppings: sliced almonds, chia seeds, fresh berries

Instructions:

- ➢ Blend blueberries, banana, almond milk, and Greek yogurt until smooth.
- ➢ Pour into a bowl and add desired toppings.

Health Benefits:

- ➢ Blueberries offer antioxidants.
- ➢ Almonds provide healthy fats and protein.
- ➢ A nutrient-packed breakfast or snack.

Preparation Time: 10 minutes

13: Baked Chicken and Vegetable Skewers

Ingredients:

- 1 pound chicken breast (cut into cubes)
- Assorted vegetables (bell peppers, cherry tomatoes, zucchini)
- 2 tablespoons olive oil
- 1 teaspoon Italian seasoning
- Salt and pepper to taste

Instructions:

- Preheat the oven to 400°F (200°C).
- Thread chicken and vegetables onto skewers.
- Mix olive oil, Italian seasoning, salt, and pepper.
- Brush the skewers with the mixture.
- Bake for 20-25 minutes or until chicken is cooked through.

Health Benefits:

- Chicken provides lean protein.
- Colorful vegetables offer vitamins and antioxidants.
- A flavorful and low-calorie option.

Preparation Time: 30 minutes

Ingredients:

- 1 cup whole wheat flour
- 1 teaspoon baking powder
- 1/2 teaspoon cinnamon
- 1 ripe banana (mashed)
- 1 cup almond milk
- 1 egg
- 1 teaspoon vanilla extract

Instructions:

- In a bowl, mix flour, baking powder, and cinnamon.
- In another bowl, whisk mashed banana, almond milk, egg, and vanilla.
- Combine wet and dry ingredients.
- Cook pancakes on a griddle until golden brown.

Health Benefits:

- Whole wheat flour adds fiber.
- Bananas provide natural sweetness.
- A wholesome and satisfying breakfast option.

Preparation Time: 20 minutes

Ingredients:

- 1 mango (diced)
- 1 can black beans (drained and rinsed)
- Red bell pepper (diced)
- Red onion (finely chopped)
- Fresh cilantro (chopped)
- Lime juice for dressing

Instructions:

- In a bowl, combine diced mango, black beans, red bell pepper, red onion, and cilantro.
- Drizzle with lime juice and toss gently.
- Serve as a refreshing salad or side dish.

Health Benefits:

- Mango provides vitamins and natural sweetness.
- Black beans offer protein and fiber.
- A light and nutrient-packed salad option.

Preparation Time: 15 minutes

16: Quinoa and Blackened Shrimp Salad

Ingredients:

- 1 cup cooked quinoa
- 1 pound shrimp (peeled and deveined)
- Cajun seasoning
- Mixed salad greens
- Cherry tomatoes (halved)
- Avocado (sliced)
- Lime vinaigrette dressing

Instructions:

- Season shrimp with Cajun seasoning.
- Sauté shrimp until blackened and cooked through.
- In a bowl, combine quinoa, mixed greens, cherry tomatoes, and avocado.
- Top with blackened shrimp.
- Drizzle with lime vinaigrette.

Health Benefits:

- Quinoa offers protein and fiber.
- Shrimp provides lean protein.
- Avocado adds healthy fats.

Preparation Time: 25 minutes

17: Sweet Potato and Chickpea Buddha Bowl

Ingredients:

- ➤ 1 large sweet potato (diced)
- ➤ 1 can chickpeas (drained and rinsed)
- ➤ Spinach leaves
- ➤ Red cabbage (shredded)
- ➤ Tahini dressing
- ➤ Pumpkin seeds for garnish

Instructions:

- ➤ Roast sweet potatoes and chickpeas in the oven.
- ➤ Arrange spinach, red cabbage, roasted sweet potatoes, and chickpeas in a bowl.
- ➤ Drizzle with tahini dressing.
- ➤ Sprinkle with pumpkin seeds.

Health Benefits:

- ➤ Sweet potatoes offer vitamins and fiber.
- ➤ Chickpeas provide protein and fiber.
- ➤ Tahini adds a creamy, nutrient-rich dressing.

Preparation Time: 30 minutes

18: Egg White Vegetable Omelette

Ingredients:

- 4 egg whites
- Spinach leaves
- Cherry tomatoes (sliced)
- Bell peppers (diced)
- Feta cheese (optional)
- Fresh herbs (such as parsley)
- Salt and pepper to taste

Instructions:

- Whisk egg whites until frothy.
- Pour into a heated non-stick skillet.
- Add spinach, cherry tomatoes, bell peppers, and feta (if using).
- Cook until set, then fold.
- Garnish with fresh herbs and season with salt and pepper.

Health Benefits:

- Egg whites provide protein.
- Vegetables offer vitamins and fiber.

➢ A low-calorie, high-protein breakfast option.

Preparation Time: 15 minutes

19: Cauliflower Fried Rice with Tofu

Ingredients:

➢ 1 cauliflower head (riced)

➢ 1 cup tofu (cubed)

➢ Mixed vegetables (peas, carrots, corn)

➢ 2 eggs (beaten)

➢ Low-sodium soy sauce

➢ Sesame oil

➢ Green onions for garnish

Instructions:

➢ Sauté tofu until golden brown.

➢ Add mixed vegetables and cauliflower rice.

➢ Push the mixture to the side and pour beaten eggs into the pan.

➢ Scramble eggs and mix with the rest of the ingredients.

➢ Season with soy sauce, sesame oil, and garnish with green onions.

Health Benefits:

> Cauliflower replaces traditional rice, reducing calories.
> Tofu provides plant-based protein.
> A flavorful and low-carb alternative.

Preparation Time: 25 minutes

20: Berry and Almond Overnight Oats

Ingredients:

> 1/2 cup rolled oats
> 1/2 cup almond milk
> Mixed berries (strawberries, blueberries, raspberries)
> 1 tablespoon almond butter
> Chia seeds for added texture

Instructions:

> In a jar, combine rolled oats and almond milk.
> Add mixed berries, almond butter, and chia seeds.
> Stir well, cover, and refrigerate overnight.
> Enjoy a quick and nutritious breakfast.

Health Benefits:

> Oats provide fiber for sustained energy.

> Berries offer antioxidants.

> Almond butter adds healthy fats.

Preparation Time: 5 minutes (plus overnight refrigeration)

21: Mediterranean Chickpea Salad

Ingredients:

> 1 can chickpeas (drained and rinsed)

> Cucumber (diced)

> Cherry tomatoes (halved)

> Red onion (finely chopped)

> Kalamata olives (sliced)

> Feta cheese (crumbled)

> Olive oil and lemon dressing

> Fresh oregano for garnish

Instructions:

> Combine chickpeas, cucumber, cherry tomatoes, red onion, olives, and feta in a bowl.

> Drizzle with olive oil and lemon dressing.

> Toss gently and garnish with fresh oregano.

Health Benefits:

- ➢ Chickpeas provide protein and fiber.
- ➢ Vegetables offer vitamins and antioxidants.
- ➢ A refreshing and satisfying salad option.

Preparation Time: 15 minutes

22: Turkey and Vegetable Stuffed Bell Peppers

Ingredients:

- ➢ 4 bell peppers (halved and seeds removed)
- ➢ Lean ground turkey
- ➢ Quinoa (cooked)
- ➢ Black beans (canned, drained, and rinsed)
- ➢ Corn kernels
- ➢ Diced tomatoes
- ➢ Taco seasoning
- ➢ Shredded cheese for topping

Instructions:

- ➢ Preheat the oven to 375°F (190°C).
- ➢ In a skillet, brown ground turkey and mix with quinoa, black beans, corn, diced tomatoes, and taco seasoning.

- ➢ Stuff bell pepper halves with the turkey mixture.
- ➢ Top with shredded cheese.
- ➢ Bake for 25-30 minutes or until peppers are tender.

Health Benefits:

- ➢ Turkey provides lean protein.
- ➢ Quinoa adds fiber and nutrients.
- ➢ Colorful vegetables offer vitamins.

Preparation Time: 40 minutes

23: Lemon Garlic Shrimp and Asparagus Stir-Fry

Ingredients:

- ➢ Shrimp (peeled and deveined)
- ➢ Asparagus spears (trimmed and cut into pieces)
- ➢ Garlic (minced)
- ➢ Lemon juice
- ➢ Low-sodium soy sauce
- ➢ Sesame oil
- ➢ Red pepper flakes (optional)
- ➢ Brown rice for serving

Instructions:

> ➤ Sauté shrimp and asparagus in a pan with garlic.
> ➤ In a bowl, mix lemon juice, soy sauce, sesame oil, and red pepper flakes.
> ➤ Pour the sauce over the shrimp and asparagus.
> ➤ Stir-fry until shrimp are cooked through.
> ➤ Serve over brown rice.

Health Benefits:

> ➤ Shrimp provides lean protein.
> ➤ Asparagus offers vitamins and fiber.
> ➤ A flavorful and low-calorie stir-fry.

Preparation Time: 20 minutes

24: Stuffed Portobello Mushrooms with Quinoa and Spinach

Ingredients:

> ➤ Portobello mushrooms (stems removed)
> ➤ Quinoa (cooked)
> ➤ Spinach leaves (sautéed)
> ➤ Cherry tomatoes (diced)
> ➤ Feta cheese (crumbled)

➢ Balsamic glaze for drizzling

➢ Fresh basil for garnish

Instructions:

➢ Preheat the oven to 375°F (190°C).

➢ In each mushroom cap, layer quinoa, sautéed spinach, diced tomatoes, and feta.

➢ Bake for 15-20 minutes.

➢ Drizzle with balsamic glaze and garnish with fresh basil.

Health Benefits:

➢ Quinoa provides protein and fiber.

➢ Spinach offers iron and vitamins.

➢ A creative and nutrient-rich dish.

Preparation Time: 30 minutes

25: Cauliflower and Broccoli Soup

Ingredients:

➢ 1 head cauliflower (florets)

➢ 2 cups broccoli florets

➢ Onion (chopped)

➢ Vegetable broth (low-sodium)

- ➢ Garlic (minced)
- ➢ Nutmeg and black pepper to taste
- ➢ Greek yogurt for garnish

Instructions:

- ➢ In a pot, sauté onions and garlic until softened.
- ➢ Add cauliflower, broccoli, and vegetable broth.
- ➢ Simmer until vegetables are tender.
- ➢ Blend until smooth.
- ➢ Season with nutmeg and black pepper.
- ➢ Garnish with a dollop of Greek yogurt.

Health Benefits:

- ➢ Cauliflower and broccoli offer vitamins and fiber.
- ➢ A comforting and low-calorie soup option.

Preparation Time: 35 minutes

26: Blackened Tilapia Tacos with Mango Salsa

Ingredients:

- ➢ Tilapia fillets
- ➢ Cajun seasoning
- ➢ Corn tortillas
- ➢ Shredded cabbage

- ➢ Mango salsa (diced mango, red onion, cilantro, lime juice)
- ➢ Greek yogurt for topping

Instructions:

- ➢ Season tilapia with Cajun seasoning and grill until cooked.
- ➢ Warm corn tortillas.
- ➢ Assemble tacos with shredded cabbage, grilled tilapia, and mango salsa.
- ➢ Top with Greek yogurt.

Health Benefits:

- ➢ Tilapia provides lean protein.
- ➢ Mango salsa offers vitamins and natural sweetness.
- ➢ A flavorful and light taco option.

Preparation Time: 25 minutes

27: Pesto Zoodles with Cherry Tomatoes

Ingredients:

- ➢ Zucchini noodles (zoodles)
- ➢ Cherry tomatoes (halved)
- ➢ Pesto sauce

➢ Pine nuts for garnish

➢ Grated Parmesan cheese (optional)

Instructions:

➢ Spiralize zucchini into noodles.

➢ Sauté zoodles and cherry tomatoes until tender.

➢ Toss with pesto sauce.

➢ Garnish with pine nuts and Parmesan cheese if desired.

Health Benefits:

➢ Zucchini provides a low-calorie pasta alternative.

➢ Pesto adds vibrant flavors without excess calories.

➢ A quick and satisfying dinner option.

Preparation Time: 15 minutes

28: Apple and Walnut Chicken Salad

Ingredients:

➢ Cooked chicken breast (shredded)

➢ Mixed salad greens

➢ Apple slices

➢ Walnuts (chopped)

➢ Feta cheese (crumbled)

- ➢ Balsamic vinaigrette dressing

Instructions:

- ➢ In a bowl, combine shredded chicken, mixed greens, apple slices, walnuts, and feta.
- ➢ Drizzle with balsamic vinaigrette.
- ➢ Toss gently and serve.

Health Benefits:

- ➢ Chicken provides lean protein.
- ➢ Apples offer fiber and natural sweetness.
- ➢ Walnuts add omega-3 fatty acids.

Preparation Time: 20 minutes

29: Lentil and Sweet Potato Curry

Ingredients:

- ➢ 1 cup lentils (rinsed and drained)
- ➢ Sweet potatoes (peeled and diced)
- ➢ Onion (chopped)
- ➢ Curry powder
- ➢ Coconut milk (light)
- ➢ Vegetable broth (low-sodium)
- ➢ Fresh cilantro for garnish

Instructions:

> - Sauté onions until translucent.
> - Add sweet potatoes, lentils, curry powder, coconut milk, and vegetable broth.
> - Simmer until lentils and sweet potatoes are tender.
> - Garnish with fresh cilantro.

Health Benefits:

> - Lentils provide protein and fiber.
> - Sweet potatoes offer vitamins and fiber.
> - A hearty and nourishing curry.

Preparation Time: 40 minutes

30: Caprese Stuffed Chicken Breast

Ingredients:

> - Chicken breasts (boneless and skinless)
> - Fresh mozzarella cheese (sliced)
> - Tomatoes (sliced)
> - Fresh basil leaves
> - Balsamic glaze for drizzling
> - Salt and pepper to taste

Instructions:

> Preheat the oven to 375°F (190°C).

> Cut a pocket into each chicken breast.

> Stuff with mozzarella, tomatoes, and basil.

> Season with salt and pepper.

> Bake for 25-30 minutes.

> Drizzle with balsamic glaze before serving.

Health Benefits:

> Chicken provides lean protein.

> Tomatoes offer vitamins and antioxidants.

> A flavorful and light dinner option.

Preparation Time: 35 minutes

31: Shrimp and Veggie Stir-Fry with Brown Rice

Ingredients:

> Shrimp (peeled and deveined)

> Broccoli florets

> Bell peppers (sliced)

> Snap peas

> Carrots (julienne)

> Low-sodium teriyaki sauce

> Brown rice (cooked)

Instructions:

> Sauté shrimp in a pan until pink.

> Add vegetables and stir-fry until crisp-tender.

> Pour low-sodium teriyaki sauce over the mixture.

> Serve over cooked brown rice.

Health Benefits:

> Shrimp provides lean protein.

> Colorful vegetables offer vitamins and fiber.

> Brown rice adds complex carbohydrates.

Preparation Time: 20 minutes

32: Chickpea and Spinach Curry

Ingredients:

> 1 can chickpeas (drained and rinsed)

> Fresh spinach leaves

> Onion (chopped)

> Garlic (minced)

> Curry powder

> Coconut milk (light)

> Vegetable broth (low-sodium)

> Basmati rice for serving

Instructions:

> Sauté onions and garlic until softened.

> Add chickpeas, curry powder, coconut milk, and vegetable broth.

> Simmer until chickpeas are heated through.

> Stir in fresh spinach until wilted.

> Serve over cooked basmati rice.

Health Benefits:

> Chickpeas provide protein and fiber.

> Spinach offers iron and vitamins.

> A flavorful and nutritious curry.

Preparation Time: 30 minutes

33: Turkey and Quinoa Stuffed Acorn Squash

> Ingredients:

> Acorn squash (halved and seeds removed)

> Lean ground turkey

> Quinoa (cooked)

> Cranberries (dried)

- ➢ Pecans (chopped)
- ➢ Maple syrup
- ➢ Cinnamon and nutmeg to taste

Instructions:

- ➢ Roast acorn squash until tender.
- ➢ Brown ground turkey and mix with quinoa, cranberries, pecans, maple syrup, cinnamon, and nutmeg.
- ➢ Stuff the squash halves with the turkey and quinoa mixture.
- ➢ Bake for an additional 15 minutes.

Health Benefits:

- ➢ Turkey provides lean protein.
- ➢ Quinoa adds protein and fiber.
- ➢ Acorn squash offers vitamins and a natural sweetness.

Preparation Time: 45 minutes

34: Teriyaki Tofu and Vegetable Skewers

Ingredients:

- ➢ Extra-firm tofu (pressed and cubed)

- ➢ Bell peppers (sliced)
- ➢ Zucchini (sliced)
- ➢ Pineapple chunks
- ➢ Low-sodium teriyaki sauce
- ➢ Brown rice for serving

Instructions:

- ➢ Marinate tofu in teriyaki sauce for 30 minutes.
- ➢ Thread tofu, bell peppers, zucchini, and pineapple onto skewers.
- ➢ Grill until vegetables are tender.
- ➢ Serve over cooked brown rice.

Health Benefits:

- ➢ Tofu provides plant-based protein.
- ➢ Vegetables offer vitamins and fiber.
- ➢ A flavorful and vegetarian option.

Preparation Time: 40 minutes

35: Cabbage and Apple Slaw with Grilled Chicken

Ingredients:

- ➢ Chicken breasts (grilled and sliced)
- ➢ Green cabbage (shredded)
- ➢ Red cabbage (shredded)
- ➢ Apple (julienned)
- ➢ Greek yogurt dressing
- ➢ Dijon mustard
- ➢ Apple cider vinegar

Instructions:

- ➢ In a bowl, combine shredded cabbages, julienned apple, and sliced grilled chicken.
- ➢ In a separate bowl, whisk together Greek yogurt, Dijon mustard, and apple cider vinegar for dressing.
- ➢ Toss the slaw with the dressing until well coated.
- ➢ Serve as a light and refreshing salad.

Health Benefits:

- ➢ Grilled chicken provides lean protein.
- ➢ Cabbages offer vitamins and fiber.

> ➢ Apples add natural sweetness.

Preparation Time: 25 minutes

36: Quinoa and Vegetable Stuffed Peppers

Ingredients:

- ➢ Bell peppers (halved and seeds removed)
- ➢ Quinoa (cooked)
- ➢ Black beans (canned, drained, and rinsed)
- ➢ Corn kernels
- ➢ Salsa
- ➢ Taco seasoning
- ➢ Shredded cheese for topping

Instructions:

- ➢ Preheat the oven to 375°F (190°C).
- ➢ Mix cooked quinoa, black beans, corn, salsa, and taco seasoning.
- ➢ Stuff the pepper halves with the quinoa mixture.
- ➢ Top with shredded cheese.
- ➢ Bake for 20-25 minutes.

Health Benefits:

- ➢ Quinoa provides protein and fiber.

- ➢ Black beans add plant-based protein.
- ➢ A colorful and flavorful dish.

Preparation Time: 35 minutes

37: Lemon Herb Chicken with Roasted Vegetables

Ingredients:

- ➢ Chicken thighs (bone-in, skin-on)
- ➢ Baby potatoes (halved)
- ➢ Carrots (cut into sticks)
- ➢ Brussels sprouts (halved)
- ➢ Lemon zest and juice
- ➢ Fresh herbs (rosemary, thyme)
- ➢ Olive oil
- ➢ Salt and pepper to taste

Instructions:

- ➢ Preheat the oven to 400°F (200°C).
- ➢ Season chicken thighs with lemon zest, lemon juice, fresh herbs, salt, and pepper.
- ➢ Arrange chicken and vegetables on a baking sheet.
- ➢ Drizzle with olive oil.

> Roast until chicken is cooked through and vegetables are golden.

Health Benefits:

> Chicken thighs provide protein.
> Colorful vegetables offer vitamins and fiber.
> A simple and wholesome one-pan meal.

Preparation Time: 45 minutes

38: Spinach and Mushroom Stuffed Chicken Breast

Ingredients:

> Chicken breasts (boneless and skinless)
> Fresh spinach leaves
> Mushrooms (sliced)
> Garlic (minced)
> Low-fat cream cheese
> Olive oil
> Italian seasoning
> Salt and pepper to taste

Instructions:

> Preheat the oven to 375°F (190°C).
> Sauté mushrooms and garlic until tender.
> Mix mushrooms with fresh spinach and cream cheese.
> Cut a pocket into each chicken breast and stuff with the spinach mixture.
> Season with Italian seasoning, salt, and pepper.
> Bake for 25-30 minutes.

Health Benefits:

> Chicken provides lean protein.
> Spinach and mushrooms offer vitamins and minerals.
> A flavorful and low-calorie stuffed chicken.

Preparation Time: 35 minutes

39: Quinoa and Black Bean Stuffed Sweet Potatoes

Ingredients:

> Sweet potatoes (baked)
> Quinoa (cooked)
> Black beans (canned, drained, and rinsed)

- ➢ Avocado (sliced)
- ➢ Salsa
- ➢ Lime wedges for garnish

Instructions:

- ➢ Cut a slit in each baked sweet potato.
- ➢ Fluff the insides with a fork.
- ➢ Mix cooked quinoa and black beans.
- ➢ Stuff sweet potatoes with the quinoa and black bean mixture.
- ➢ Top with sliced avocado, salsa, and a squeeze of lime.

Health Benefits:

- ➢ Sweet potatoes offer vitamins and fiber.
- ➢ Quinoa provides protein and fiber.
- ➢ Avocado adds healthy fats.

Preparation Time: 30 minutes

40: Broccoli and Cheddar Stuffed Chicken Roll-Ups

Ingredients:

- ➢ Chicken breasts (pounded thin)
- ➢ Broccoli florets (steamed)
- ➢ Cheddar cheese (shredded)
- ➢ Dijon mustard
- ➢ Garlic powder
- ➢ Paprika
- ➢ Salt and pepper to taste

Instructions:

- ➢ Preheat the oven to 375°F (190°C).
- ➢ Spread Dijon mustard on each pounded chicken breast.
- ➢ Layer with steamed broccoli and cheddar cheese.
- ➢ Roll up each chicken breast and secure with toothpicks.
- ➢ Season with garlic powder, paprika, salt, and pepper.
- ➢ Bake for 25-30 minutes.

Health Benefits:

- ➢ Chicken provides lean protein.
- ➢ Broccoli offers vitamins and fiber.
- ➢ A cheesy and satisfying dish.

Preparation Time: 35 minutes

CONCLUSION

Embarking on a weight loss journey after pregnancy is not just about shedding pounds; it's a holistic commitment to nourishing your body, reclaiming your well-being, and embracing a healthier lifestyle for both you and your little one.

The "Weight Loss After Pregnancy Cookbook" is designed not only to guide you through delicious and nutritious recipes but to inspire a sustainable approach to postpartum wellness.

Remember, this is a transformative journey that goes beyond the kitchen. It's about making mindful choices, fostering self-love, and embracing the incredible resilience of your body.

Each recipe in this cookbook is a step towards a stronger, healthier you, combining flavors that delight the palate with ingredients that nourish from within.

As you savor the wholesome meals crafted with care, may you find joy in the process, celebrate every achievement, and appreciate the incredible strength you possess.

This cookbook is not just a collection of recipes; it's a companion on your path to a balanced, fulfilling, and vibrant life post-pregnancy.

May these recipes empower you to make choices that align with your health goals, fostering a positive relationship with food and wellness.

Here's to embracing the journey, savoring the flavors, and achieving the balance that promotes lasting well-being.

Your health is an investment, and this cookbook is a guide to making that investment a flavorful and nourishing success.

Cheers to your journey of post-pregnancy wellness!